HOW-TO-GUIDE: ALDARA (IMIQUIMOD)

Navigating the Challenges of Rare Skin Disorders

Dr. Gabi Hugo

Contents

CHAPTER ONE

Overview of Aldara

(Imiquimod)

Imiquimod is a topical drug sold under the trade name Aldara and is employed in dermatology for treating a number of diseases. Its main role is to change the activity of the immune system to help the body attack abnormally developed skin tissues. Aldara is clearly described here: what it is, how it works, where it is used, how it is applied, and some of the possible side effects.

How it Works

The active substance forming Aldara is called imiquimod, and this medication belongs to the immune response modifiers. This applies through an activation of toll-like receptor 7 (TLR7) hence boosting the immunity system cells. It subsequently sets off several immune reactions such as the production of cytokines like interferon-alpha. These cytokines are effective in improving the recognition of previously damaged or infected tissues. Immuno-stimulation is the principal means by which

Aldara works when treating certain skin diseases, and is absolutely critical to the product's operation.

Administration and Dosage

Imiquimod has two main formulations in the market, the cream and the gel; Aldara is the trade name for Imiquimod cream Imiquimod is indicated for the treatment of various skin diseases including, genital warts, basal cell carcinoma, and actinic keratosis.

 This is because the medication, when applied correctly, and as prescribed, has dramatically helped patients suffering from viruses, especially PV and SK, without adverse effects. Thus, staying on the schedule of each disease, handling the dosage properly if missed, and seeking help from healthcare providers, patients are able to treat actinic keratosis, superficial basal cell carcinoma, and genital or perianal warts using Aldara. Patient compliance with instructions and the schedule of regular check-ups are essential

elements for getting the desired

outcomes with this medication.

Benefits of Aldara

(Imiquimod)

Aldara is also used in skin

disorders and hence is described

to be offering non-surgical

solutions for these cases. This is rather beneficial for those patients who do not like going through invasive procedures. It is done in order not to undertake surgery, use cryotherapy or laser in the removal of skin tags. This can be done at the comfort of one's home thus minimizing the need of going to the clinic often.

 Aldara is used in a treatment of actinic keratosis, a precancerous skin disease and some superficial basal cell carcinoma – a form of skin cancer. In the case of actinic keratosis, Aldara's application helps to avoid the further evolution of precancerous growths into skin invasive cancer. Indeed, for the superficial basal cell carcinoma, Aldara is an opportunity to treat this type of cancer without severe operations.

In its mode of operation, Aldara affects the body's immune

system by increasing its activity on abnormal or infected cells. Aldara strengthens the patient's immune system especially in regards to skin growths that are considered to be abnormal and skin infections. It is also widely used because it helps the immune system make a concentrated attack on the spot affected by the disease.

Aldara is prescribed for the external treatment of genital warts and perianal warts that are caused by HPV.

It also gives an option that is less invasive compared to cryotherapy or surgical excision. Besides, this procedure is useful in the removal of warts and may also prevent re-emergence of the growths.

CHAPTER TWO

Alternatives

Although Aldara (Imiquimod) is a good solution for some skin diseases, there are many options available based on the diagnosis and patient's preferences. Such other alternatives include other topical treatments, surgeries, and other higher level dermatological remedies. This choice should depend on the nature and degree of the disease or disorder, the patient's state, and the outcome of previous therapy. It is crucial to reach out to a qualified medical practitioner in order to find out the best suitable plan dependent on the various factors encountered.

Common Side Effects

Despite the fact that Aldara (Imiquimod) is associated with the possibility of outstanding results for treating different types of skin diseases, it is crucial to study possible side effects and have proper approach to their minimization. Mild skin reactions include moderate redness, itching, and dryness of the skin; while severe skin reactions include ulceration of the skin or formation of blisters. Consequent actions on the systemic level are not very frequent but are still possible. Thus, it is possible to minimize side effects and get maximal efficacy in using Baclofen with the right approach to its application, regular monitoring of the condition, and timely consultation with a healthcare provider. If you have any of the above severe or persisting symptoms seeks the attention of a doctor for appropriate management.

Negative Interactions

Imiquimod does not interfere with other drugs because it has low systemic bioavailability.

The external interactions are with other topical agents in the case of Aldara (Imiquimod), skin care products, and UV radiation.

Appropriate care cover entails

not utilizing products that may trigger irritation on the same area, refraining from sun exposure on the treated area and consulting a doctor whenever other treatments are being applied. Patients should always disclose the usage of all medications and products to their doctors for safer and more efficient treatment. If you develop any other effects or if your reactions to the medications change in any way, contact your healthcare professional.

Potential Errors to Be Avoided When Using Aldara (Imiquimod)

1. The side effects can include severe skin irritation, redness, or ulceration of the skin area where the lotion is applied. They also influence the outcome by having correct or incorrect application

regarding the treatment. Try as much as possible to maintain the recommended interval and time of applying the solution. Bleomycin is usually used based on the relevance of scales, normally it is used a few times a week, and changes in this schedule can occur only under the permission of a doctor.

2. If Aldara is applied to lesions that are on the areas that possess broken, irritated, or inflamed skin, the condition becomes worse and side effects worsened. Always make sure that the skin

that is to be subjected to the application of the gel is healthy and has no cuts. It is recommended not to use the cream in case you or the treated person has open wounds, cuts, or other irritated areas at the time of application.

3. Local effects may be more severe if MCP applied excessively; such as redness, swelling, or even ulceration. Using it in bigger amounts than required instead does not benefit and it can lead to side effects which would have been avoided. Therefore, ensure that you

spread a little amount of this on the affected region in accordance with the recommendations that were given. One should not exceed the prescribed level since it will not enhance the performance and might lead to certain side-effects.

4. Inadequate rinsing off the drug after the required time or improper washing of hands after use of the drug.

5. Discontinuation of the treatment as soon as initial manifestations are alleviated can cause the relapse of the

condition or incomplete regression of the lesion. Therefore, patients should continue to have the treatment as advised even when the symptoms of the infection have cleared out. You should always discuss your plans for any modification to your lifestyle or

treatment with your doctor.

When to see a doctor

Understanding when to seek the attention of a medical doctor is of utmost importance as a doctor would give you the right directives to enable you to use the medication appropriately in order to achieve the desired skin result. Endeavor to seek the attention of a medical doctor whenever you experience any reactions or side effects during the course of usage of the medication.

THE END